Let's get fit!

Name _____________ Height _________ Weight _________

Arm L _________ R _________

Chest

Waist _________

Hips _________

Thigh L _________ R _________

Calf L _________ R _________

Starting stats

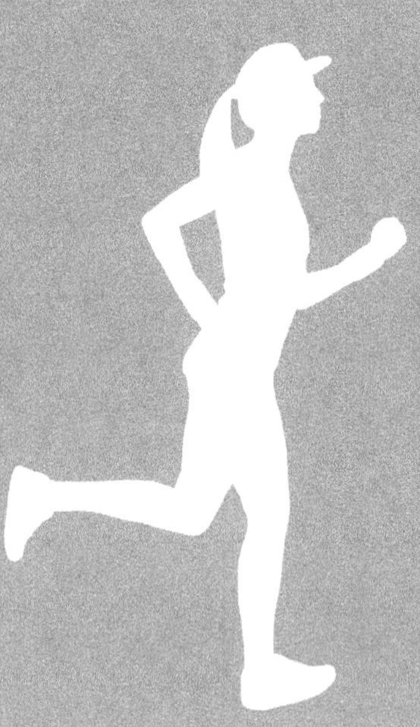

Run toward your goal
today!
Remember,
there is no change where
there is no action.

Start

Put your picture
here

Me today _______
date

Week One

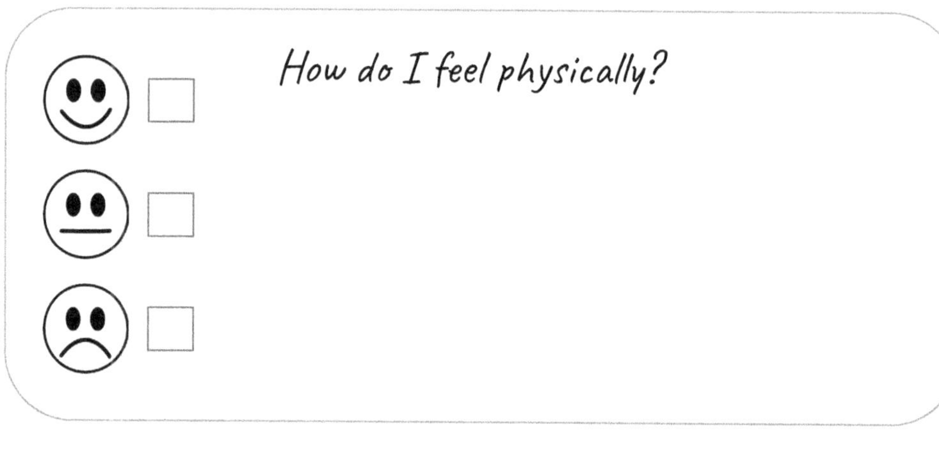

This week's GOALS

Day 1

Date _______________

breakfast

lunch

snacks

dinner

Workout

cardio ☐

☐ strength

flexibility ☐

☐ rest day

Day 2

Date _______________

breakfast

lunch

snacks

dinner

Day 3

Date ______________________

breakfast

lunch

snacks

dinner

Day 4

Date _______________

breakfast

lunch

snacks

dinner

Day 5

Date _______________

breakfast

lunch

snacks

dinner

Day 6

Date ______________________

breakfast   lunch

snacks   dinner

Workout

cardio ☐   ☐ strength

flexibility ☐   ☐ rest day

Day 7

Date ___________________

breakfast

lunch

snacks

dinner

Week one completed !

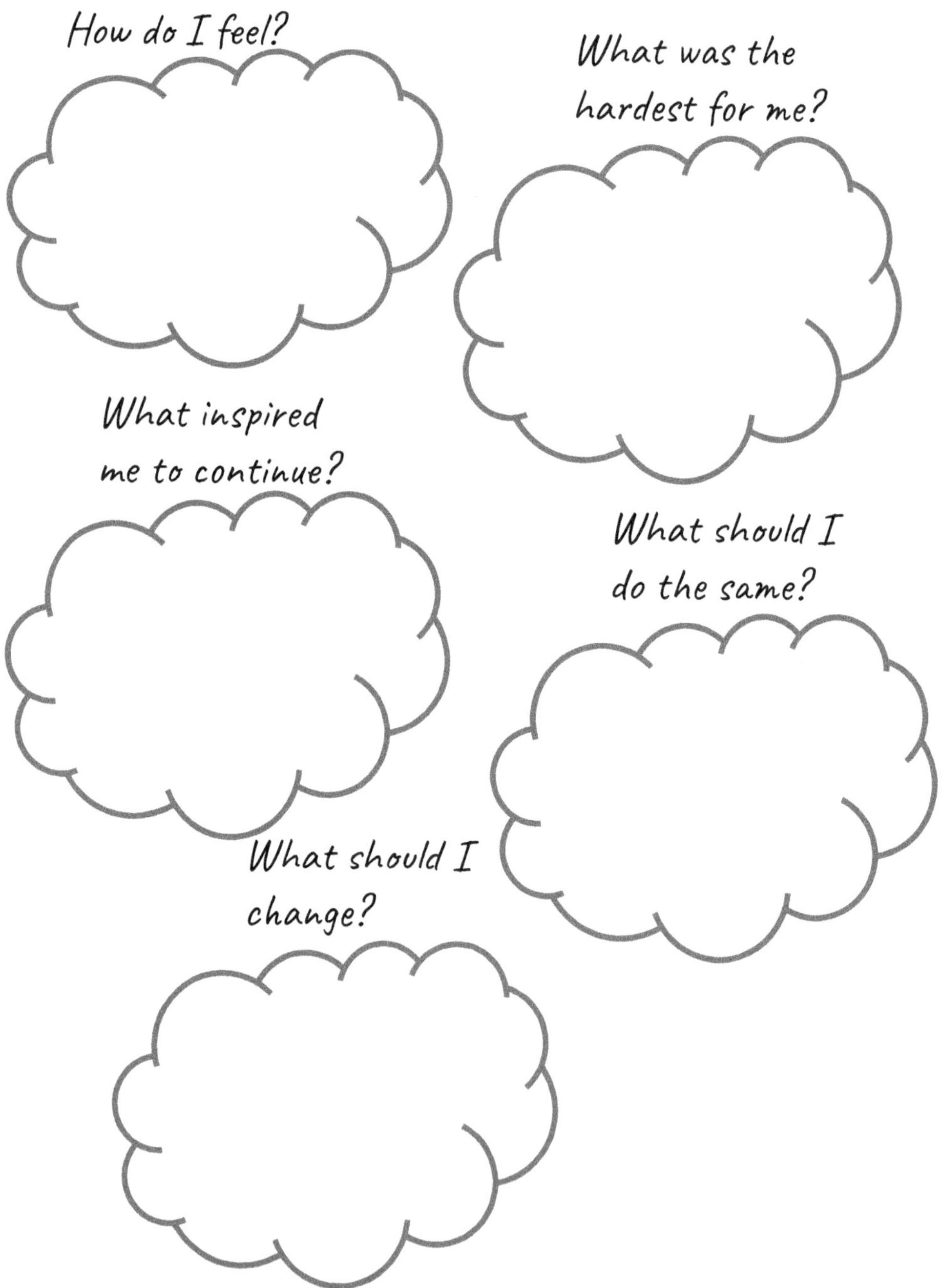

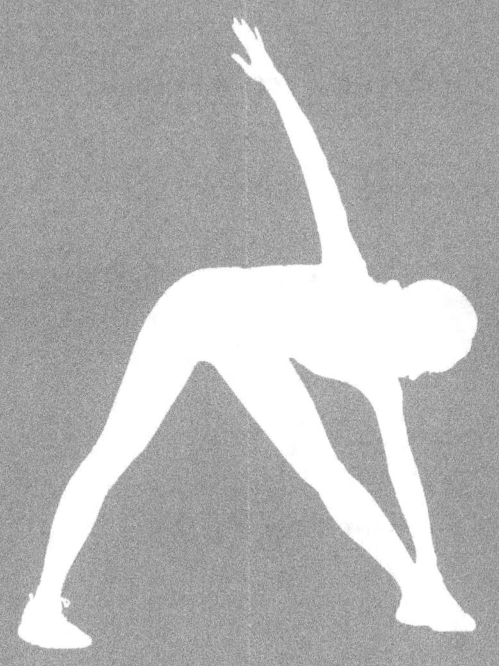

When you feel like
QUITTING
think about WHY you
STARTED

Week Two

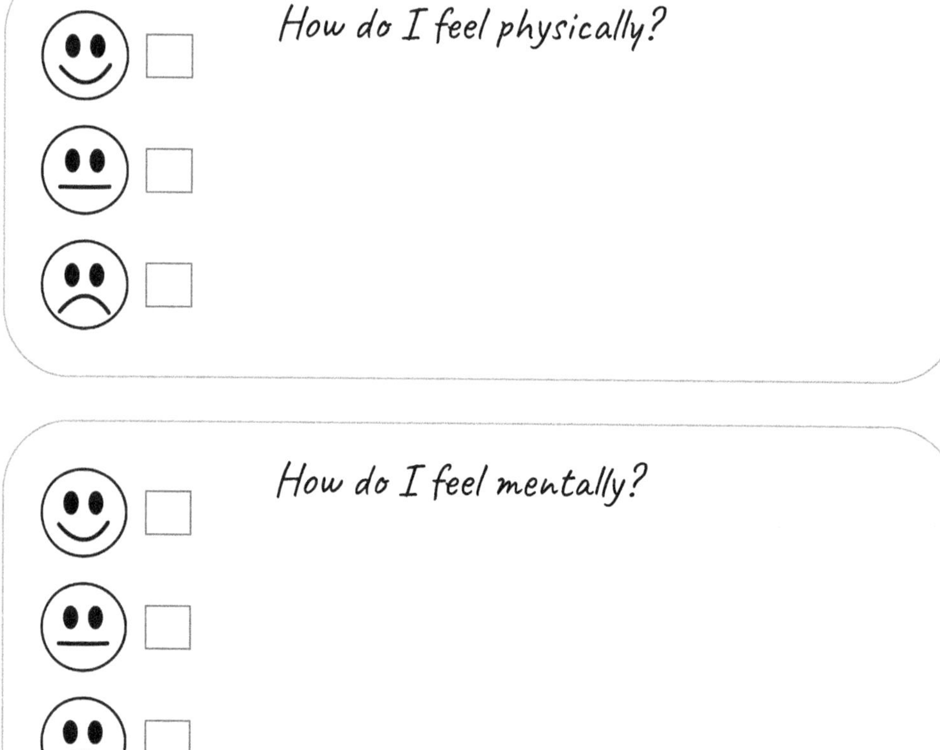

This week's GOALS

Day 8

Date _______________

breakfast

lunch

snacks

dinner

Day 9

breakfast

lunch

snacks

dinner

Workout

cardio ☐ ☐ strength

flexibility ☐ ☐ rest day

Day 10

Date ______________________

breakfast

lunch

snacks

dinner

Day 11

Date ______________________

breakfast

lunch

snacks

dinner

Day 12

Date ______________________

breakfast

lunch

snacks

dinner

Workout

cardio ☐   ☐ strength

flexibility ☐   ☐ rest day

zZzz

Day 13

Date _______________

breakfast

lunch

snacks

dinner

Day 14

Date ___________________

breakfast

lunch

snacks

dinner

Week two completed !

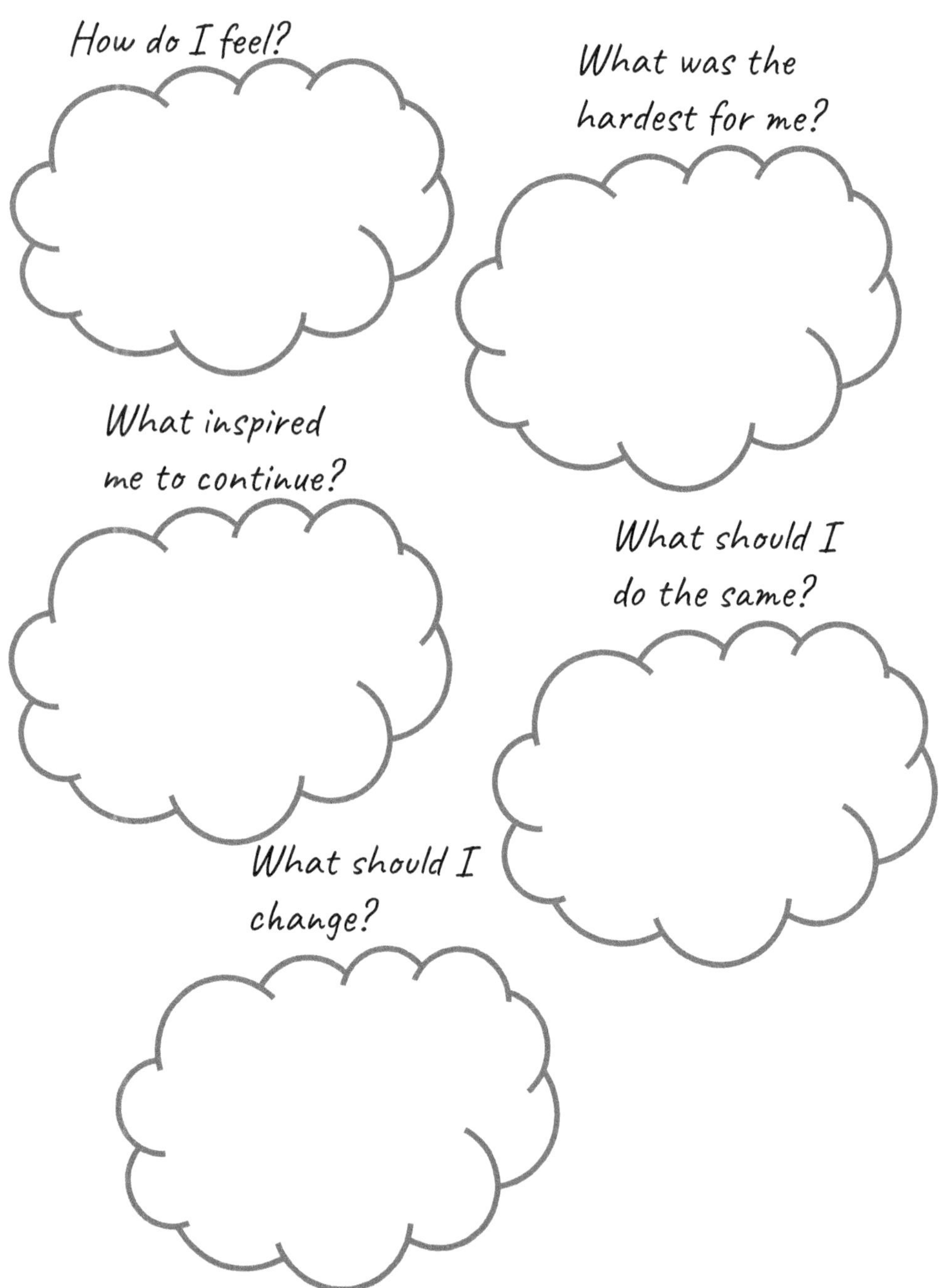

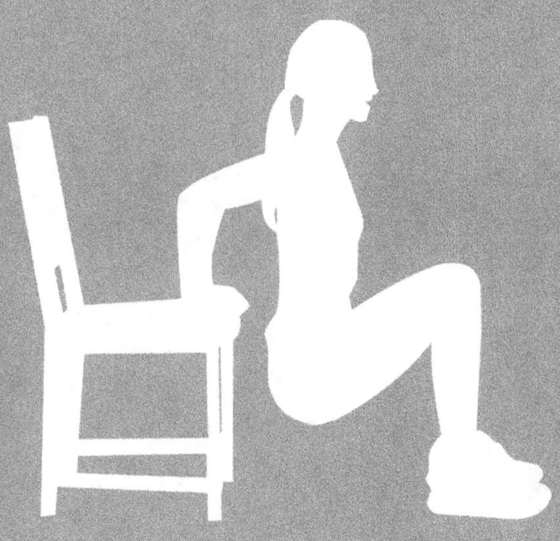

You may not be there YET.
But you're CLOSER than
YESTERDAY

Week Three

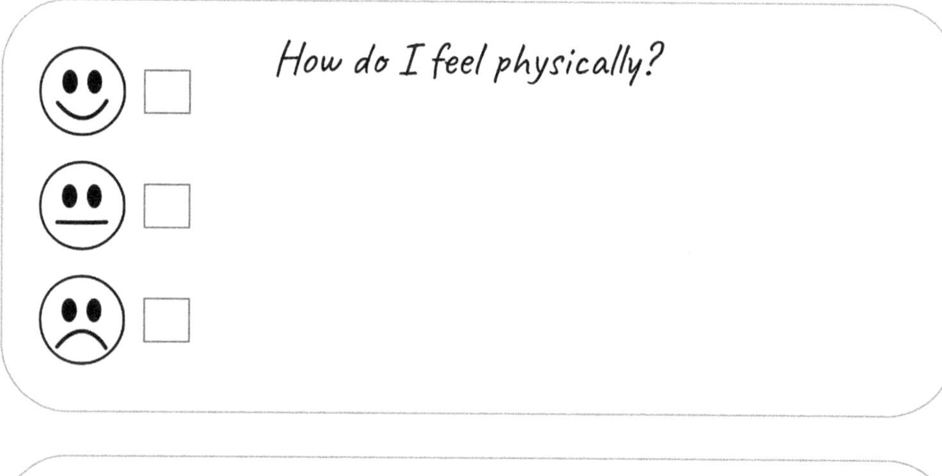

This week's GOALS

Day 15

Date ______________________

breakfast

lunch

snacks

dinner

cardio ☐ ☐ strength

flexibility ☐ ☐ rest day

Day 16

Date _______________

breakfast

lunch

snacks

dinner

Day 17

Date _______________

breakfast

lunch

snacks

dinner

Workout

cardio ☐ ☐ strength

flexibility ☐ ☐ rest day

zZzz

Day 18

Date ____________________

breakfast

lunch

snacks

dinner

Day 19

Date _______________

breakfast

lunch

snacks

dinner

Day 20

Date ___________________

breakfast

lunch

snacks

dinner

Day 21

Date ______________________

breakfast

lunch

snacks

dinner

Week three completed !

How do I feel?

What was the
hardest for me?

What inspired
me to continue?

What should I
do the same?

What should I
change?

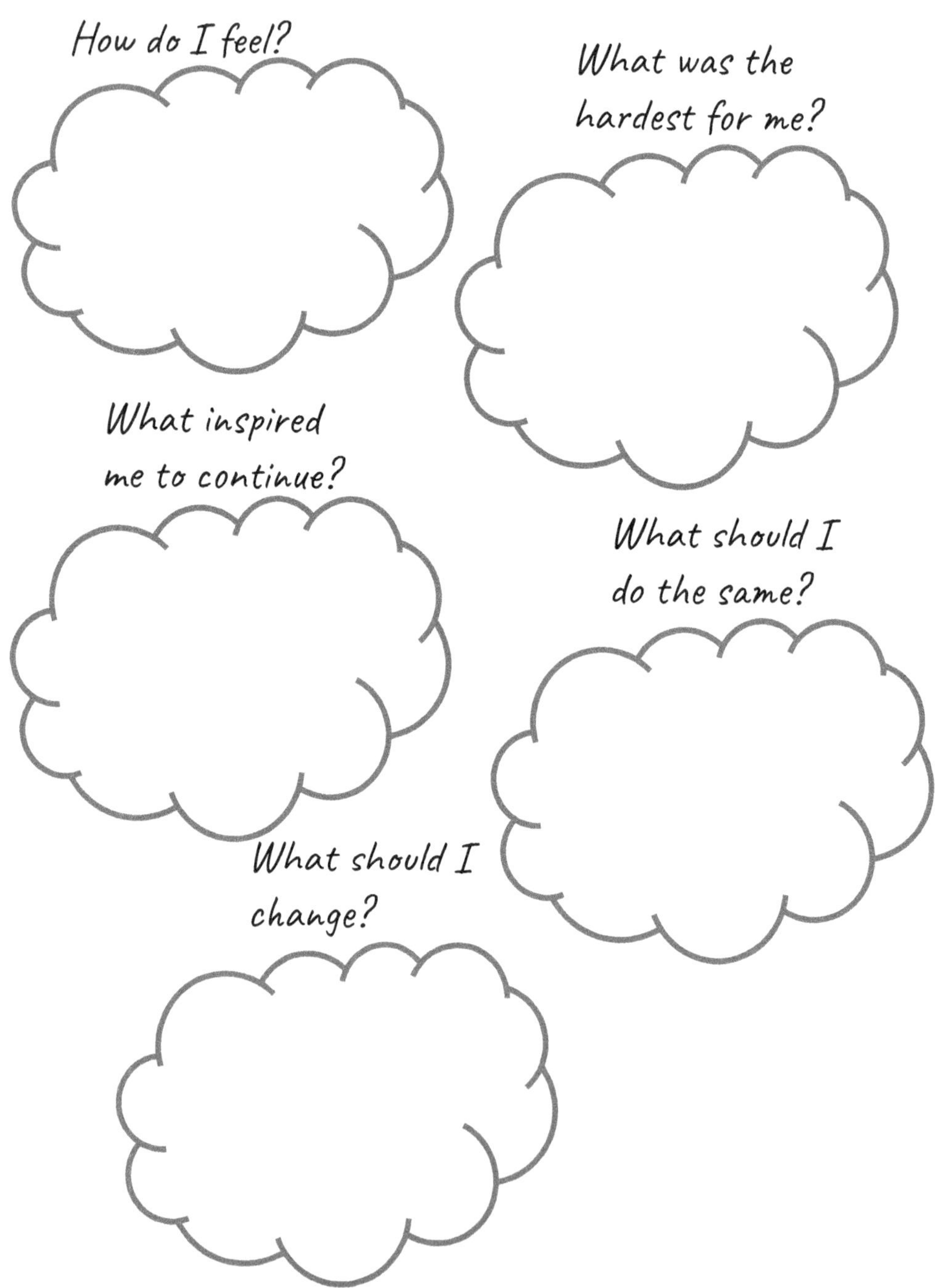

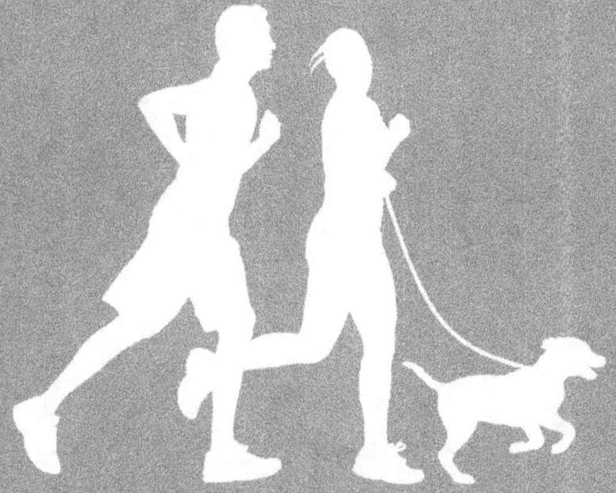

SUCCESS doesn't come from what you do OCCASIONALLY, it comes from what you do CONSISTENTLY

Week Four

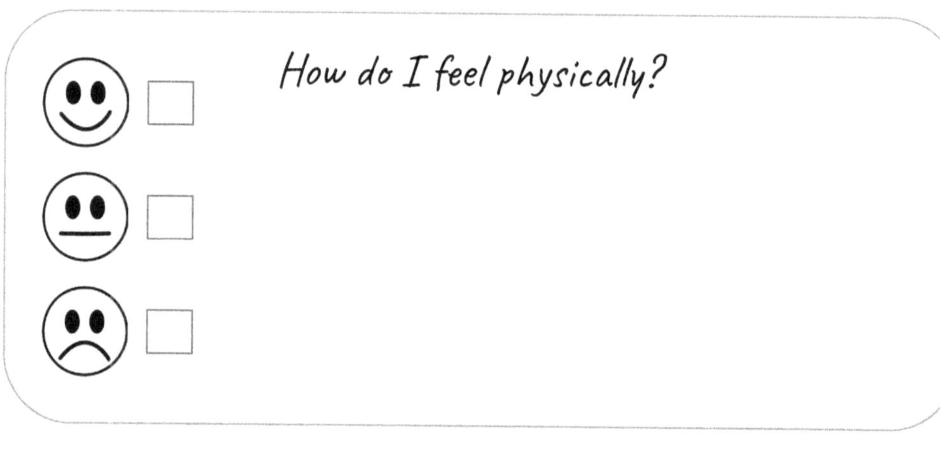

This week's GOALS

Day 22

Date ___________________

breakfast

lunch

snacks

dinner

Day 23

Date ___________________

breakfast

lunch

snacks

dinner

Day 24

Date _______________

breakfast

lunch

snacks

dinner

Day 25

breakfast

lunch

snacks

dinner

Workout

cardio ☐　☐ strength

flexibility ☐　☐ rest day

zZzz

Day 26

Date ___________________

breakfast

lunch

snacks

dinner

Day 27

Date ______________

breakfast

lunch

snacks

dinner

Day 28

Date _______________

breakfast

lunch

snacks

dinner

Week four completed !

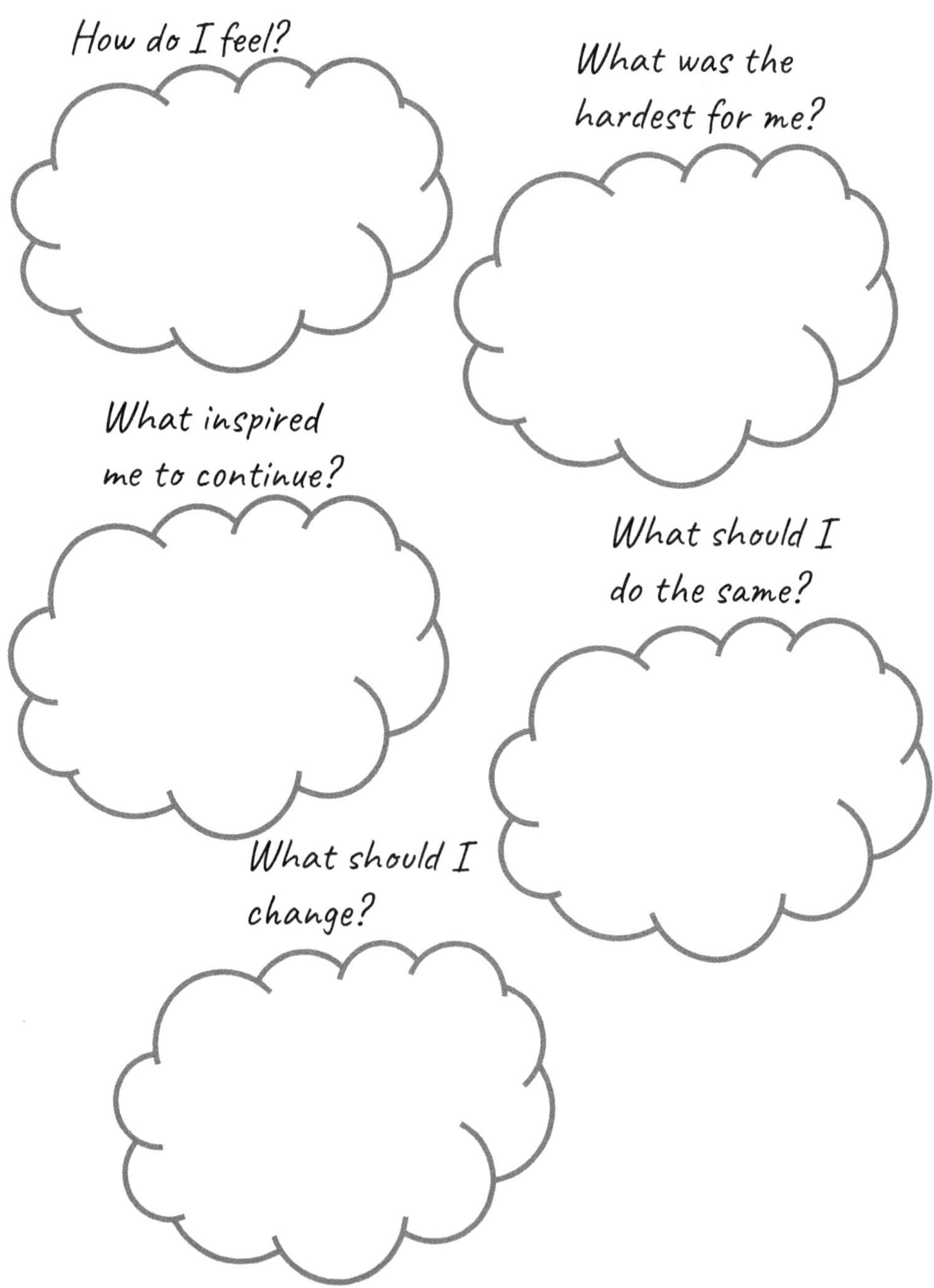

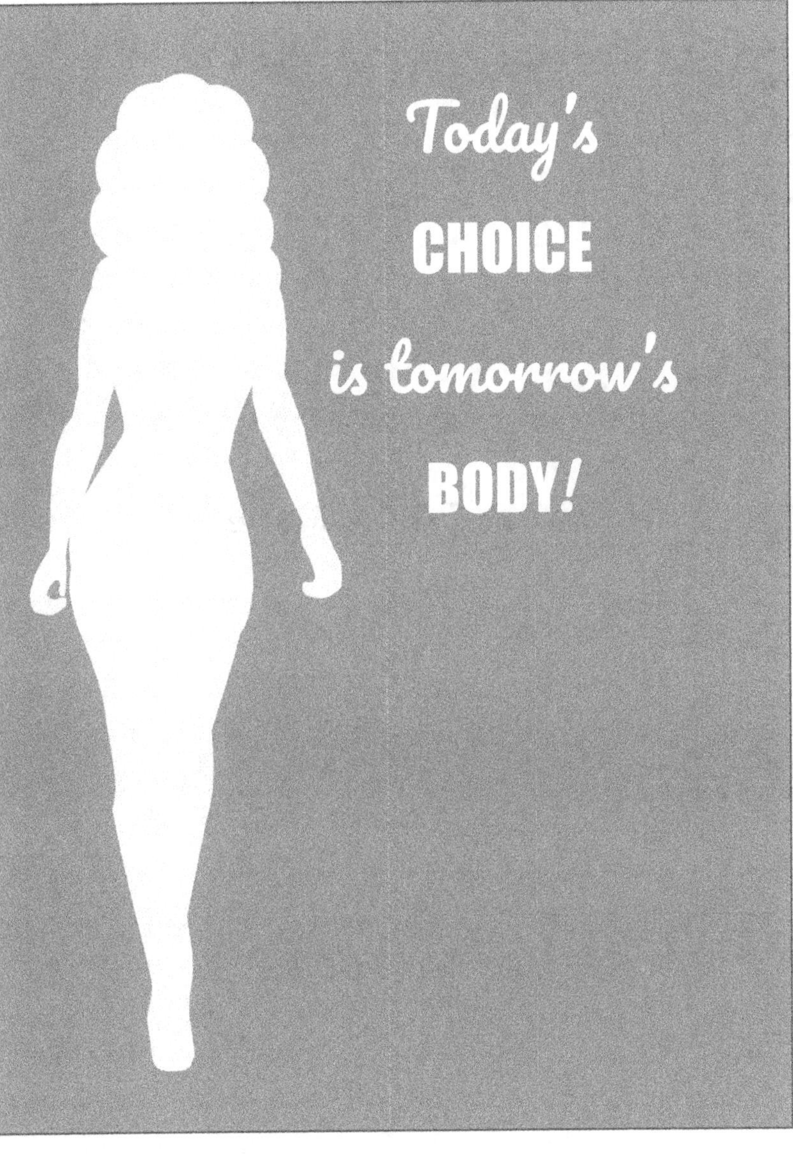

Today's
CHOICE
is tomorrow's
BODY!

Week Five

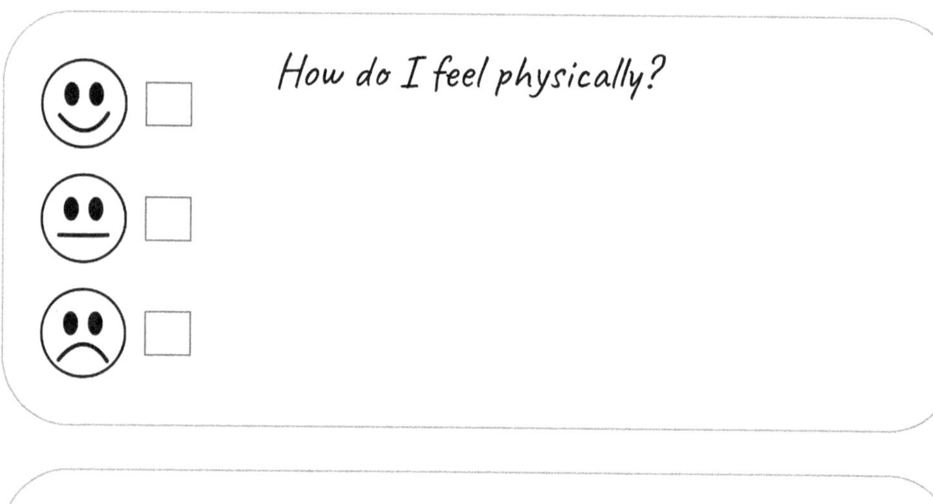

This week's GOALS

Day 29

Date _______________

breakfast

lunch

snacks

dinner

Day 30

Date ________________

breakfast

lunch

snacks

dinner

Workout

cardio ☐ ☐ strength

flexibility ☐ ☐ rest day

zZzz

Day 31

Date ___________________

breakfast

lunch

snacks

dinner

Workout

cardio ☐ ☐ strength

flexibility ☐ ☐ rest day

zZzz

Day 32

Date ______________

breakfast

lunch

snacks

dinner

Workout

cardio ☐   ☐ strength

flexibility ☐   ☐ rest day

zZzz

Day 33

Date _______________

breakfast

lunch

snacks

dinner

Day 34

Date ______________________

breakfast

lunch

snacks

dinner

Day 35

Date _______________

breakfast

lunch

snacks

dinner

Week five completed !

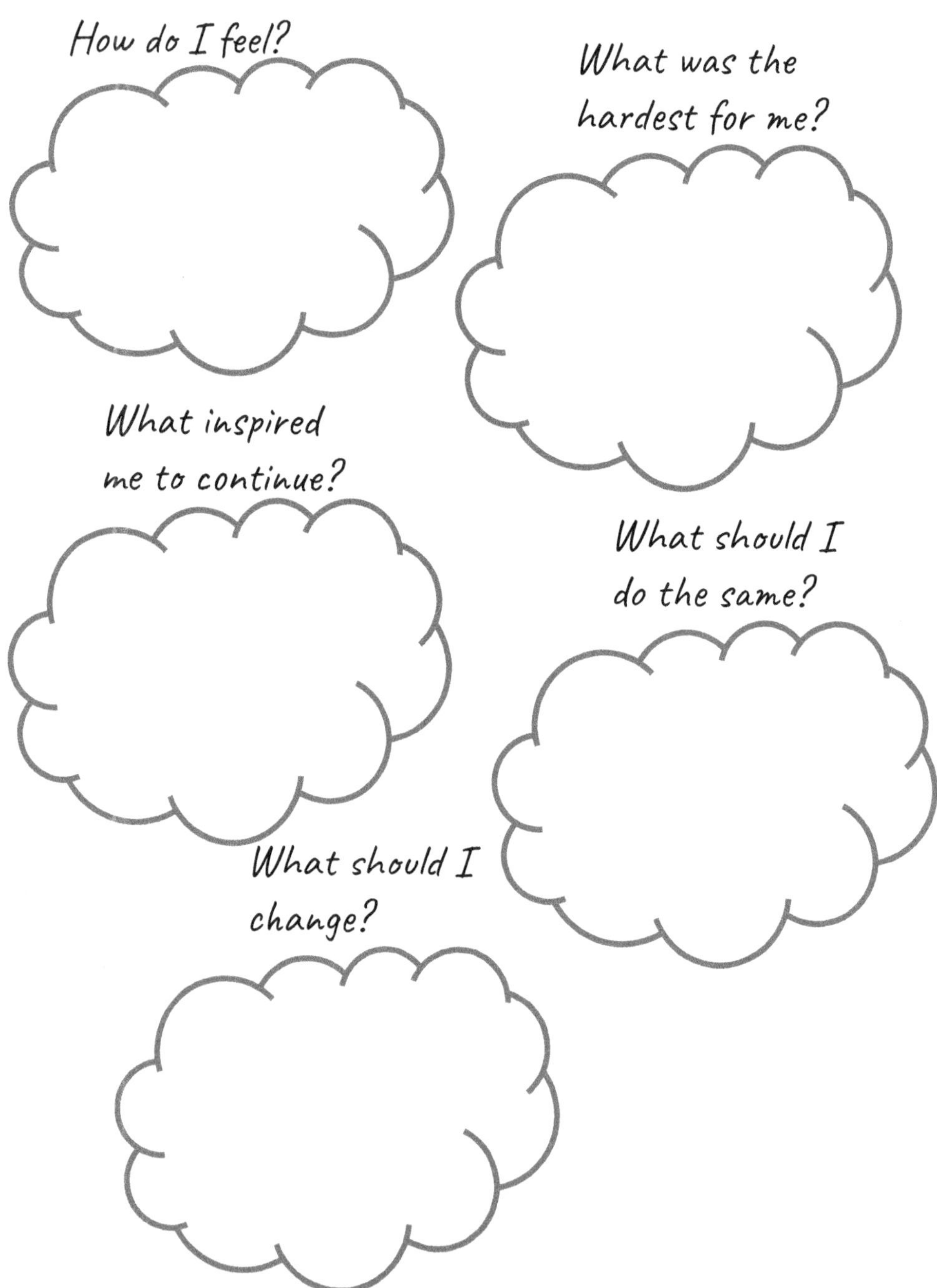

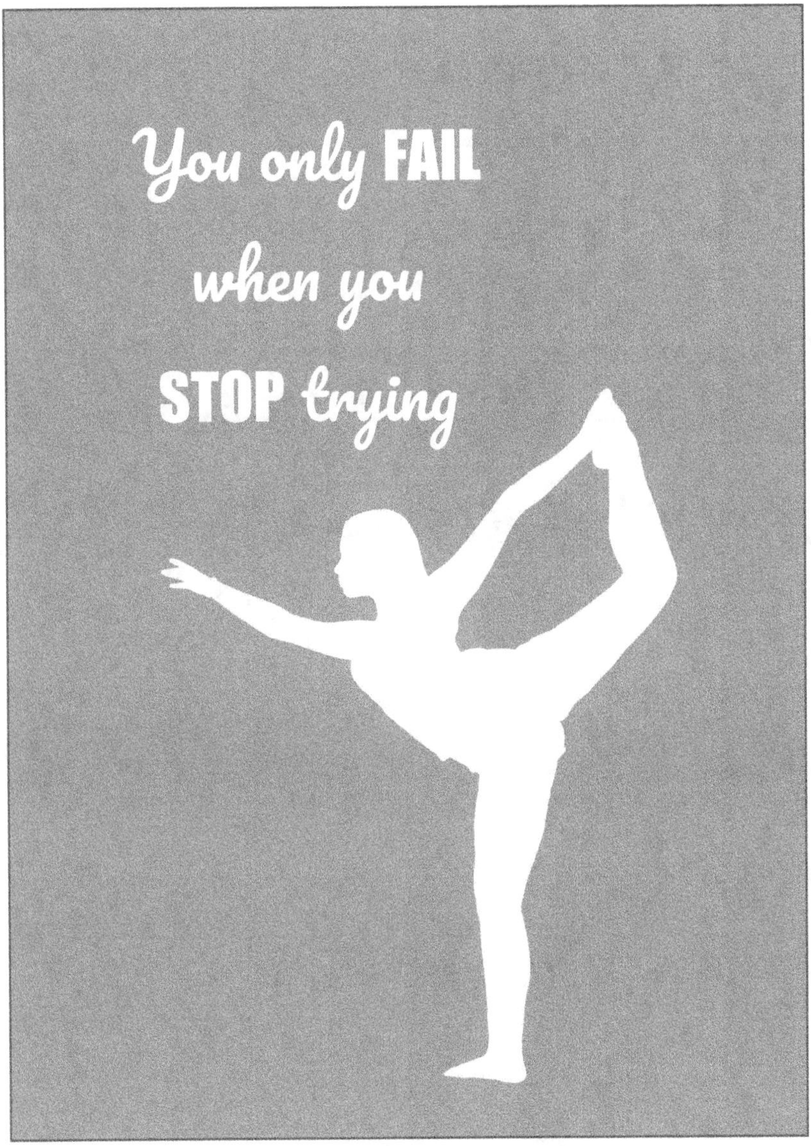

You only FAIL
when you
STOP trying

Week Six

How do I feel physically?

How do I feel mentally?

This week's GOALS

Day 36

Date _______________

breakfast

lunch

snacks

dinner

Workout

cardio ☐ ☐ strength

flexibility ☐ ☐ rest day

zZzz

Day 37

Date ________________

breakfast

lunch

snacks

dinner

Day 38

Date _______________

breakfast

lunch

snacks

dinner

Day 39

Date _______________

breakfast

lunch

snacks

dinner

Day 40

Date ___________________

breakfast

lunch

snacks

dinner

Day 41

Date _______________

breakfast

lunch

snacks

dinner

Day 42

Date _______________

breakfast

lunch

snacks

dinner

Week six completed !

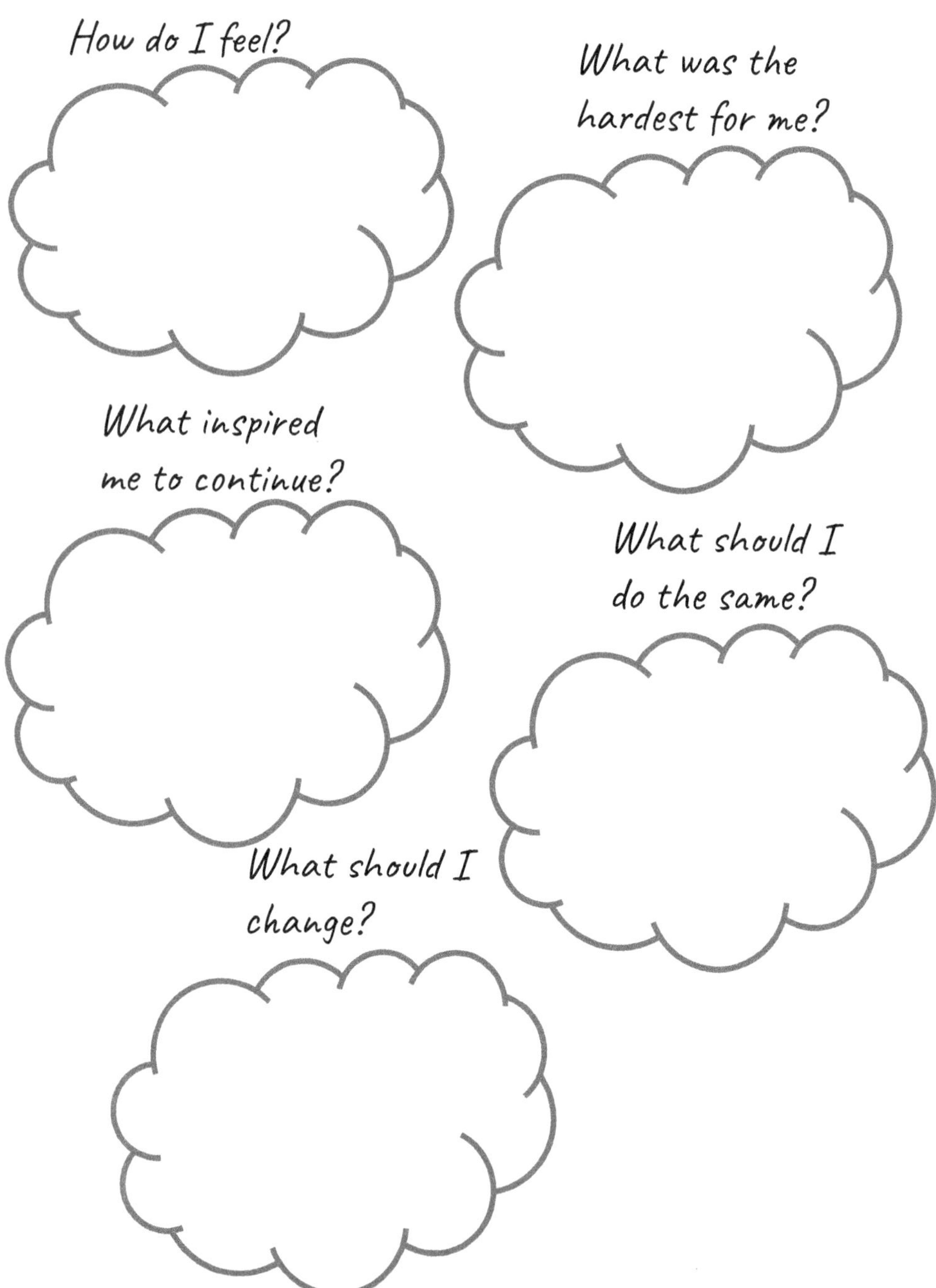

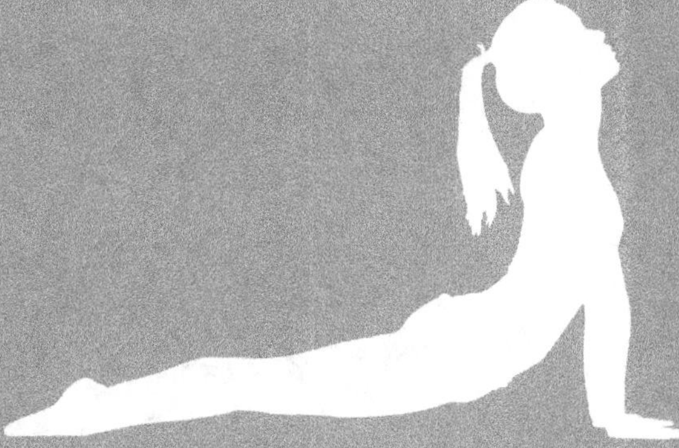
PERSEVERE
The day
you plant the SEED
is not the day
you eat the FRUIT

Week Seven

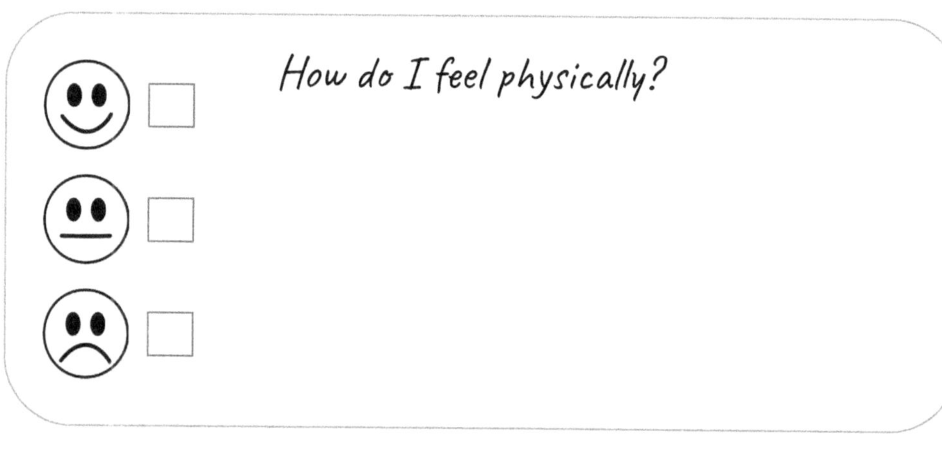

How do I feel physically?

How do I feel mentally?

This week's GOALS

Day 43

Date _______________

breakfast

lunch

snacks

dinner

Day 44

Date _______________

breakfast

lunch

snacks

dinner

Day 45

Date ___________________

breakfast

lunch

snacks

dinner

Day 46

Date _______________

breakfast

lunch

snacks

dinner

Day 47

Date _______________

breakfast

lunch

snacks

dinner

Workout

cardio ☐ ☐ strength

flexibility ☐ ☐ rest day

Day 48

Date ______________

breakfast

lunch

snacks

dinner

Day 49

Date ______________________

breakfast

lunch

snacks

dinner

Week seven completed !

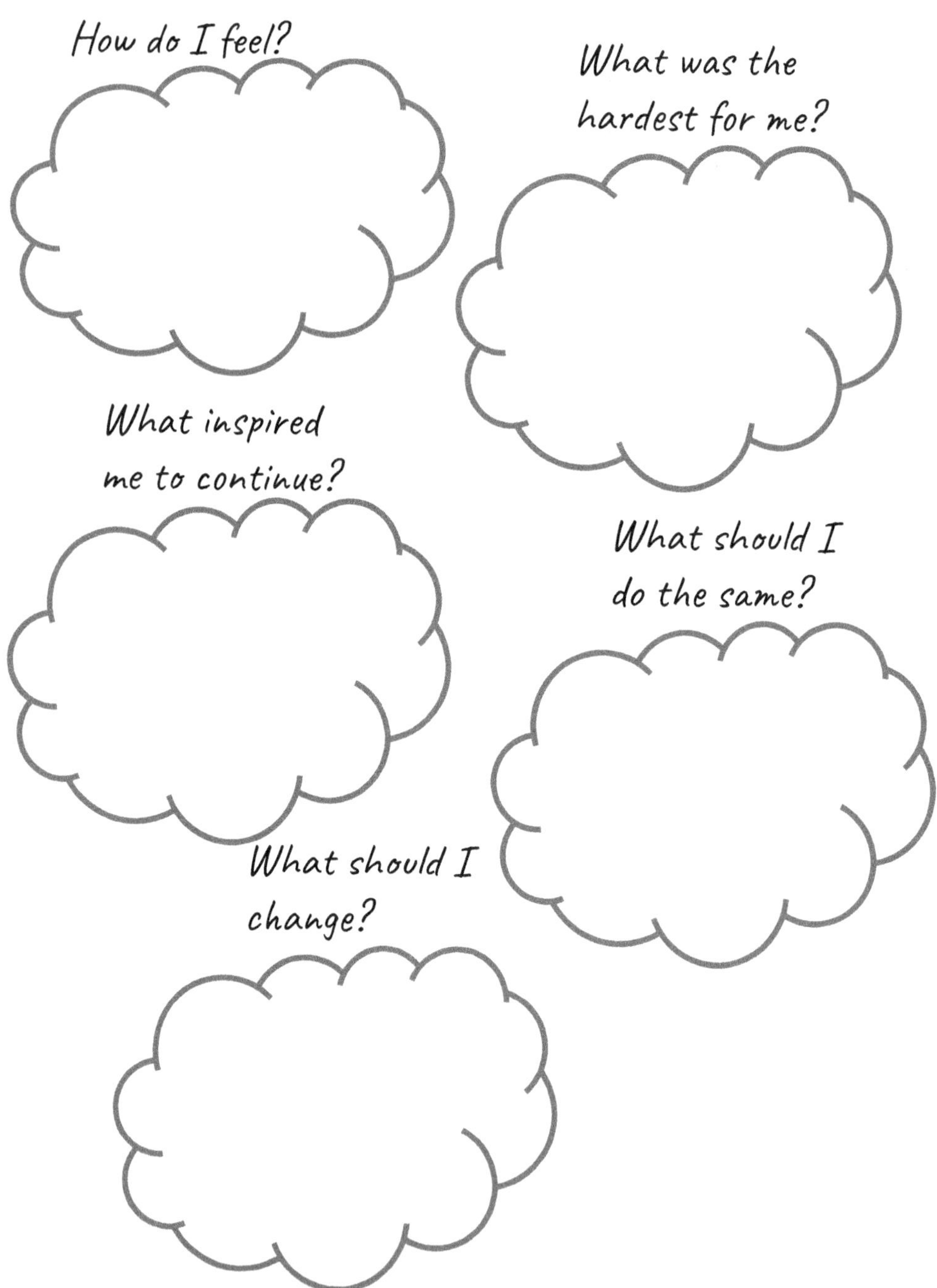

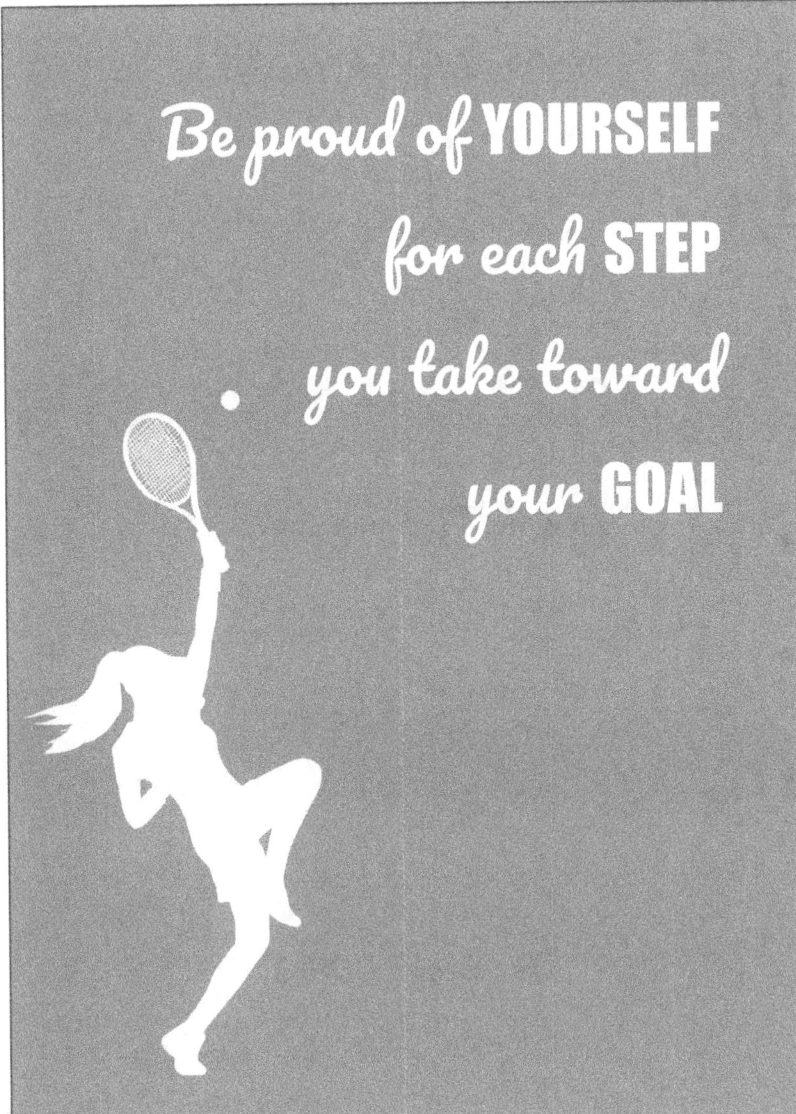

Be proud of YOURSELF
for each STEP
you take toward
your GOAL

Week Eight

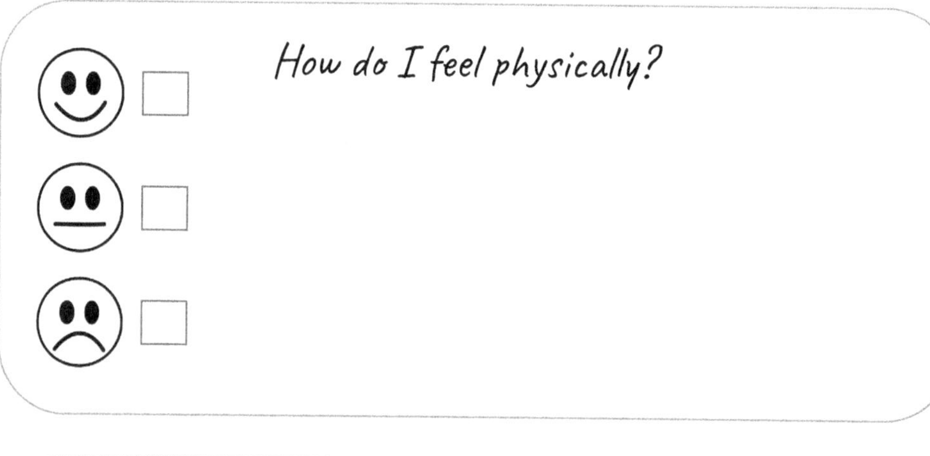

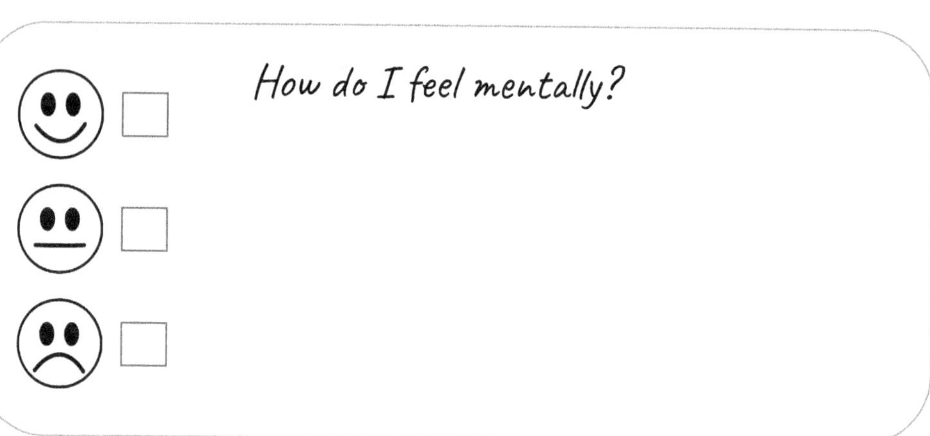

This week's GOALS

Day 50

Date ___________________

breakfast

lunch

snacks

dinner

Day 51

Date _______________

breakfast

lunch

snacks

dinner

Day 52

Date ___________________

breakfast

lunch

snacks

dinner

Day 53

Date _______________

breakfast

lunch

snacks

dinner

Workout

cardio ☐ ☐ strength

flexibility ☐ ☐ rest day

zZzz

Day 54

Date ______________________

breakfast

lunch

snacks

dinner

Day 55

Date

breakfast

lunch

snacks

dinner

Day 56

Date _______________

breakfast

lunch

snacks

dinner

Week eight completed !

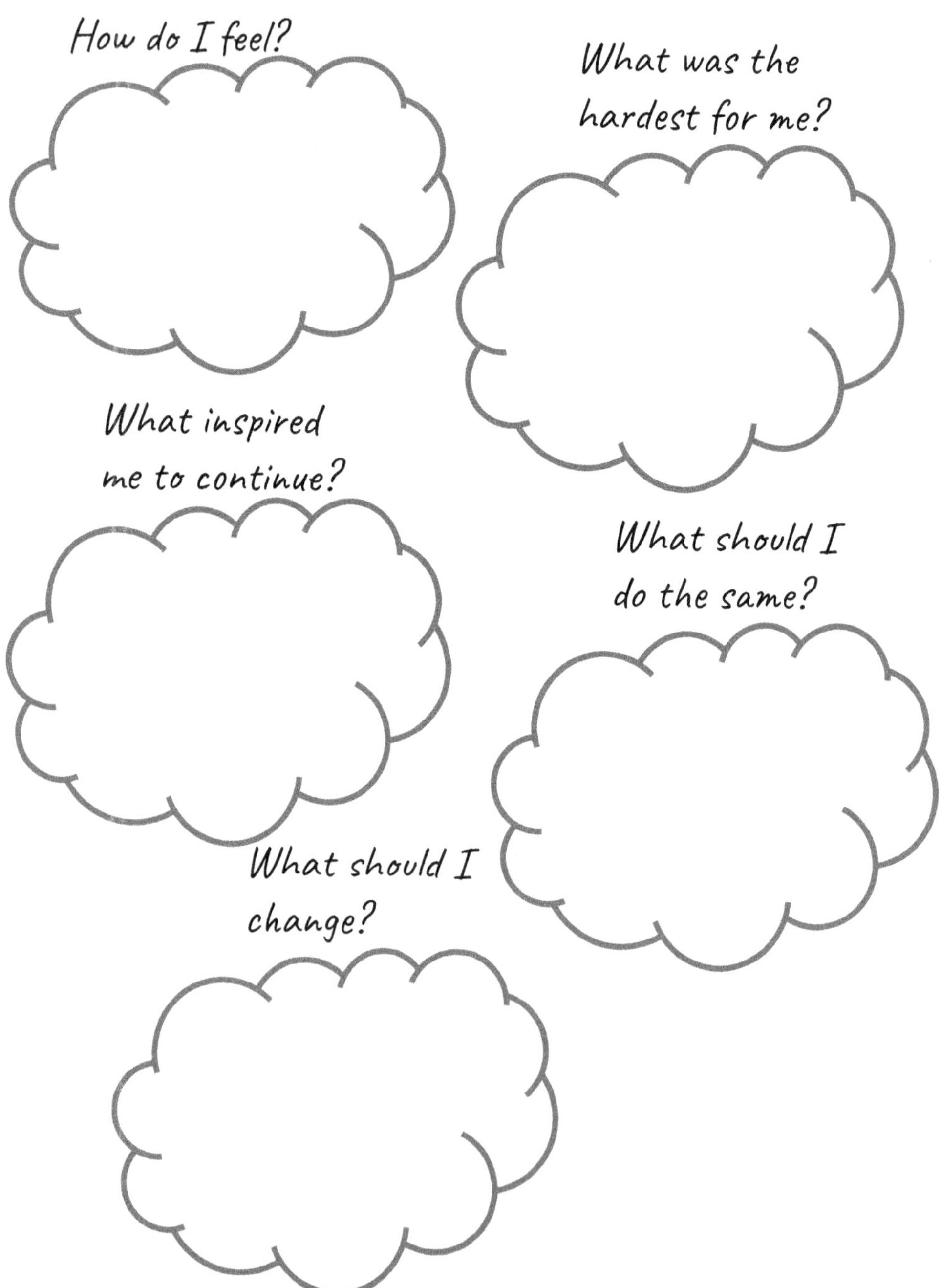

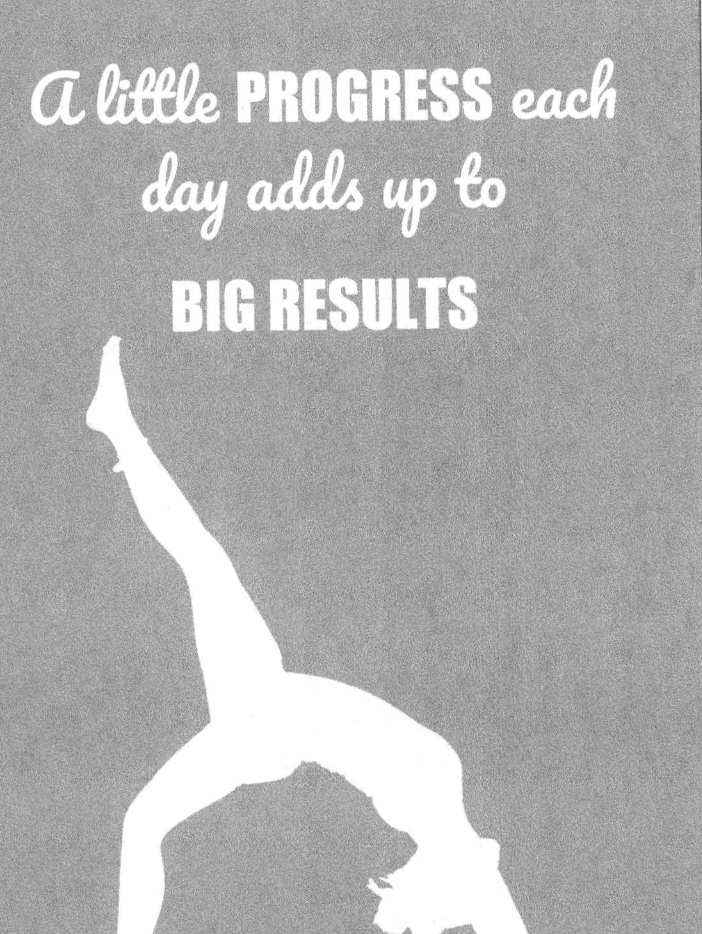
A little PROGRESS each day adds up to
BIG RESULTS

Week Nine

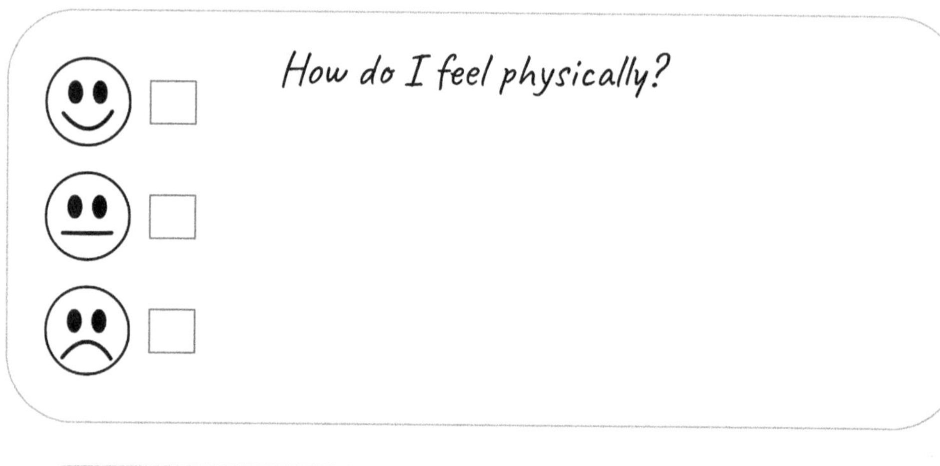

How do I feel physically?

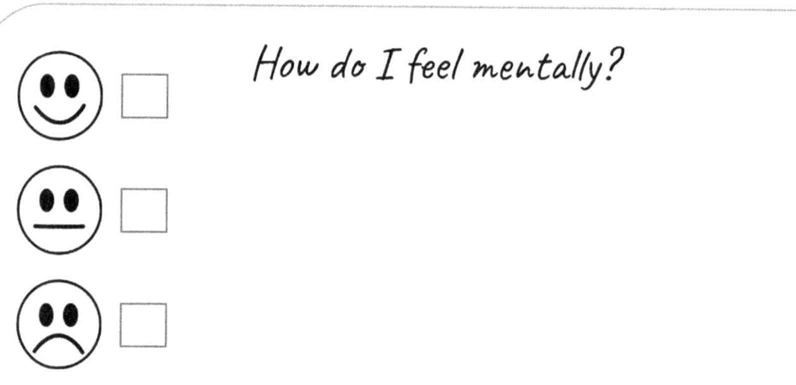

How do I feel mentally?

This week's GOALS

Day 57

Date ___________________

breakfast

lunch

snacks

dinner

Day 58

breakfast

lunch

snacks

dinner

Day 59

Date ___________________

breakfast

lunch

snacks

dinner

Day 60

Date _______________

breakfast

lunch

snacks

dinner

Day 61

Date ______________________

breakfast

lunch

snacks

dinner

Day 62

Date ___________________

breakfast

lunch

snacks

dinner

Workout

cardio ☐   ☐ strength

flexibility ☐   ☐ rest day

zZzz

Day 63

Date ___________________

breakfast

lunch

snacks

dinner

Week nine completed !

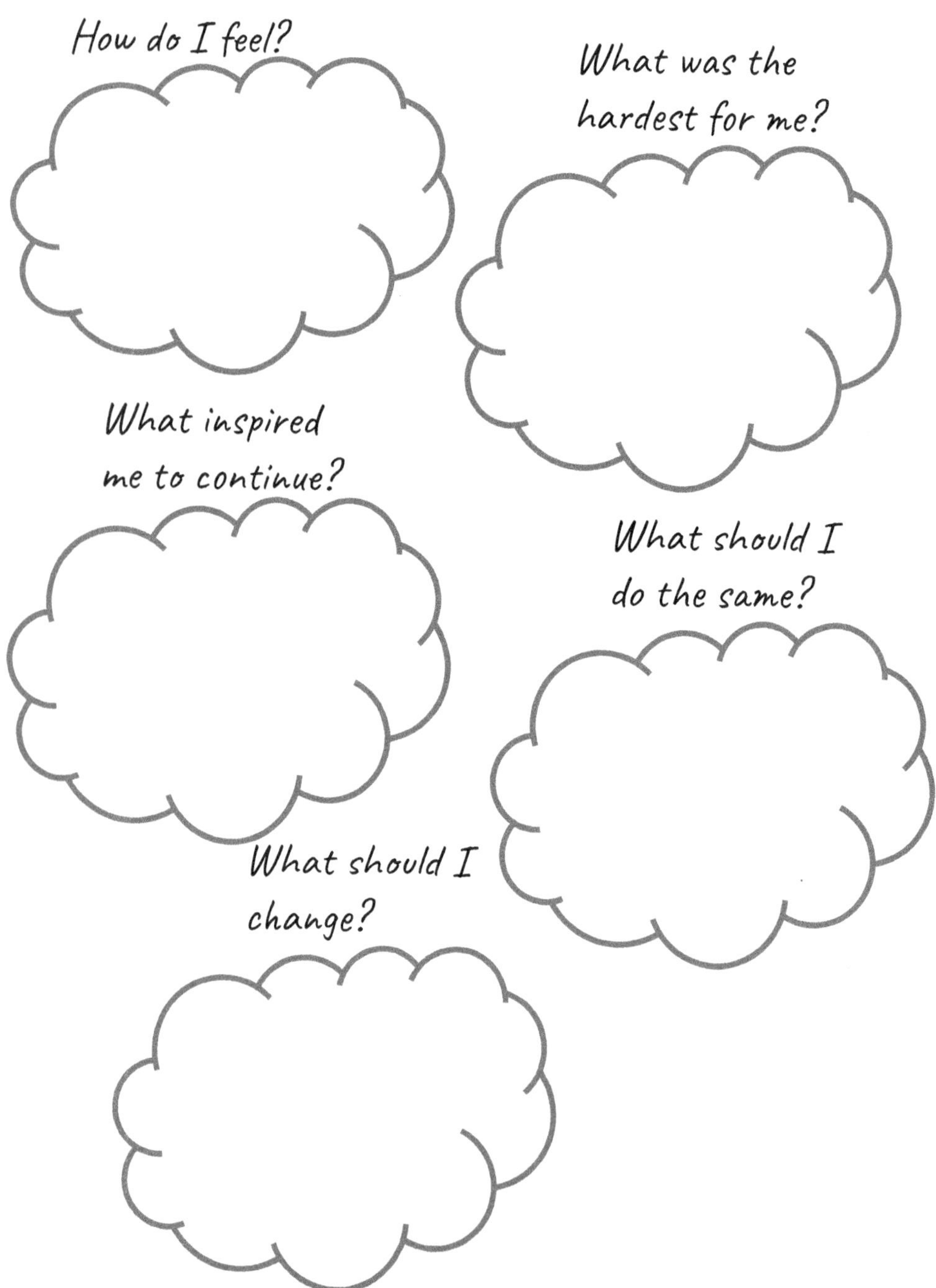

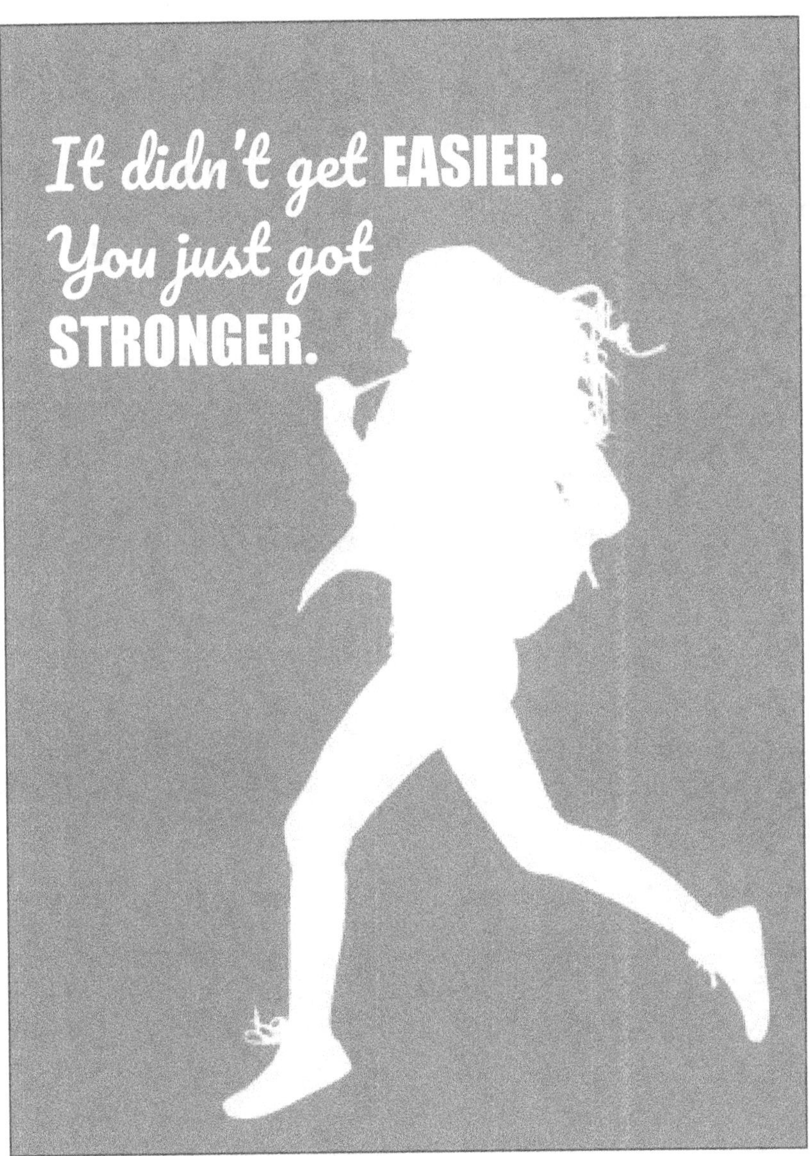It didn't get EASIER.
You just got STRONGER.

Week Ten

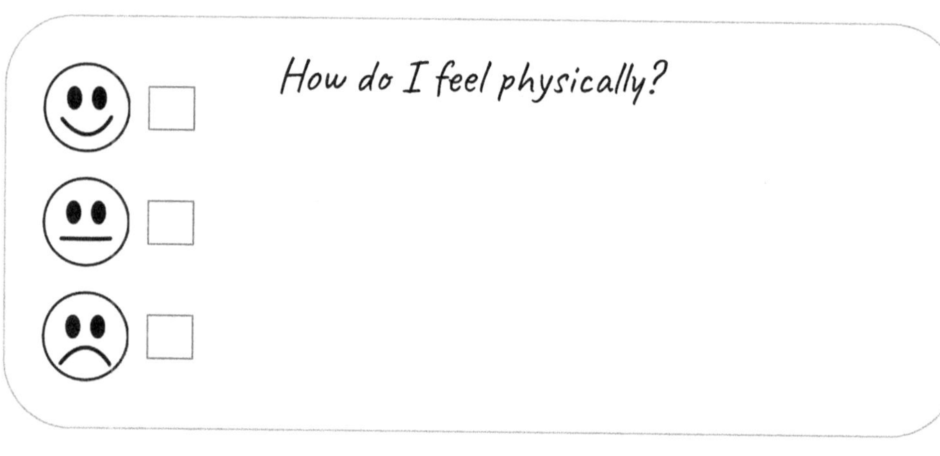

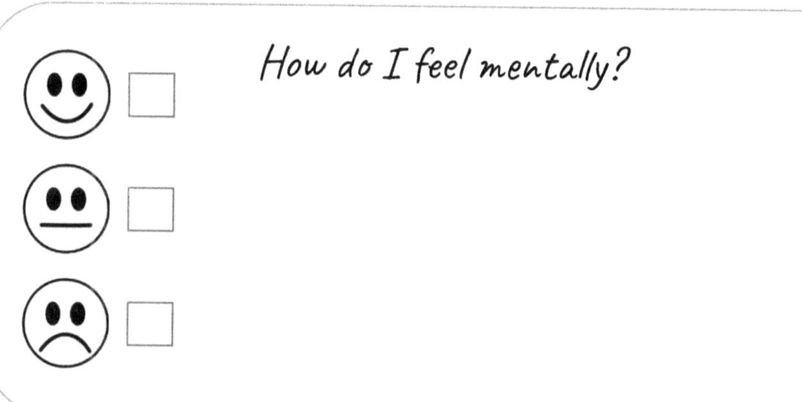

This week's GOALS

Day 64

Date _______________

breakfast

lunch

snacks

dinner

Workout

cardio ☐ ☐ strength

flexibility ☐ ☐ rest day

zZzz

Day 65

Date ______________________

breakfast

lunch

snacks

dinner

Day 66

Date ___________________

breakfast

lunch

snacks

dinner

Workout

cardio ☐ ☐ strength

flexibility ☐ ☐ rest day

zZzz

Day 67

Date ______________________

breakfast

lunch

snacks

dinner

Day 68

Date ______________

breakfast

lunch

snacks

dinner

Day 69

Date _______________

breakfast

lunch

snacks

dinner

Day 70

Date _______________

breakfast

lunch

snacks

dinner

Week ten completed !

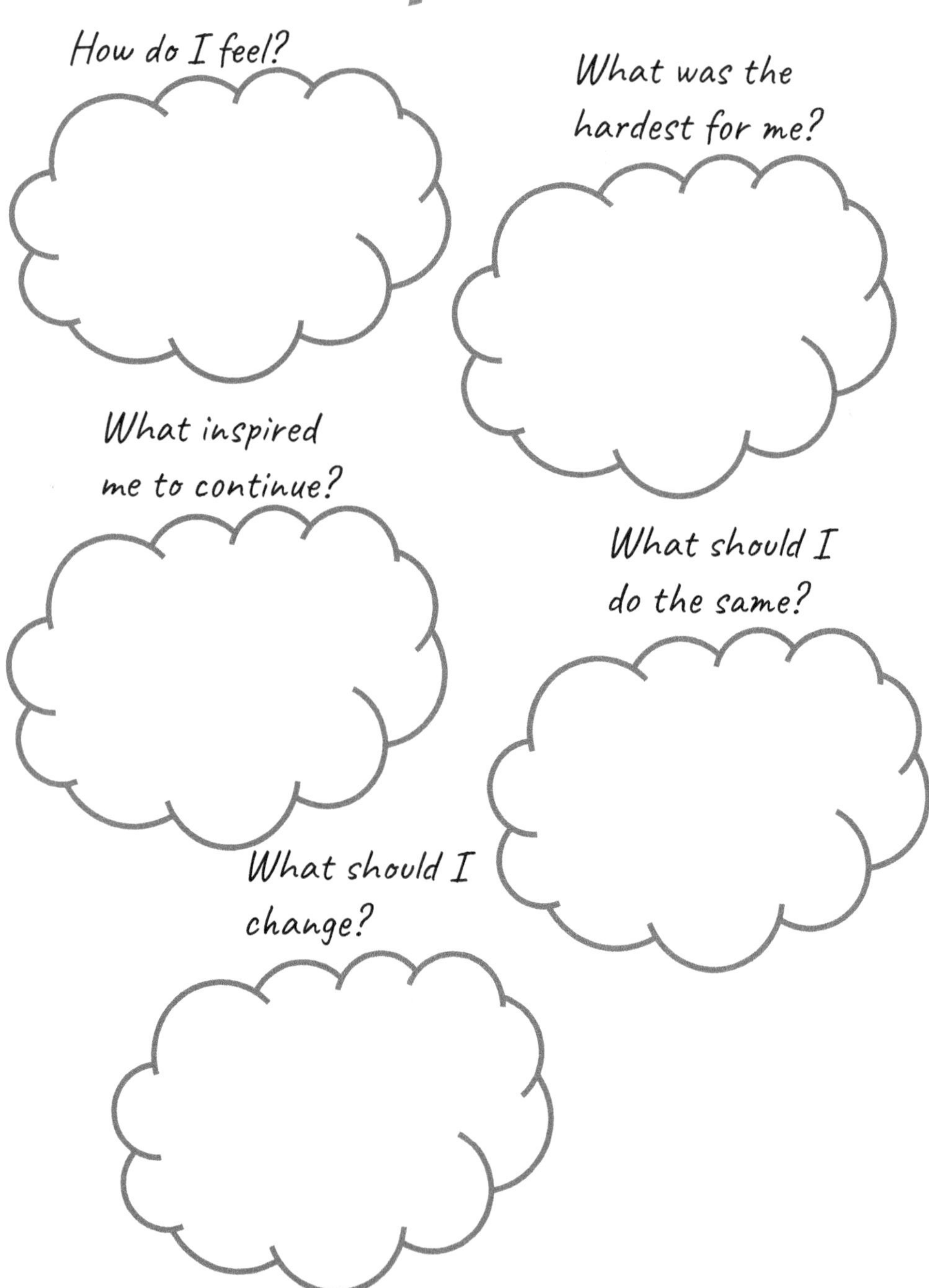

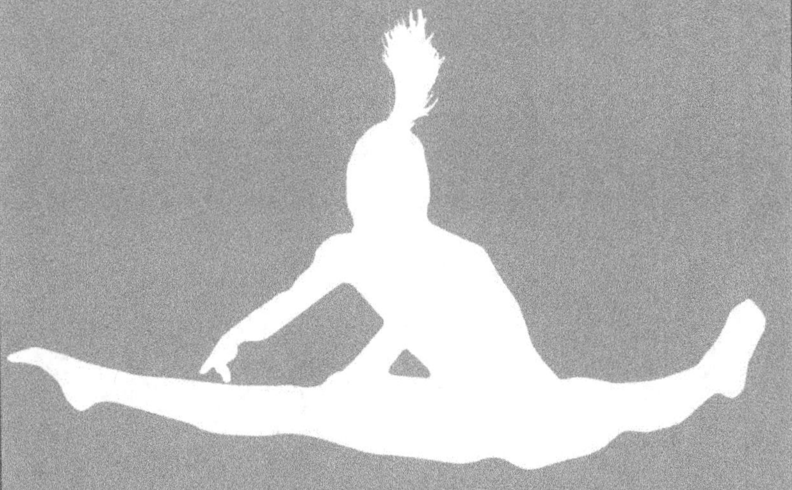

Your body can do almost ANYTHING.
It's your MIND
that you have to CONVINCE.

Week Eleven

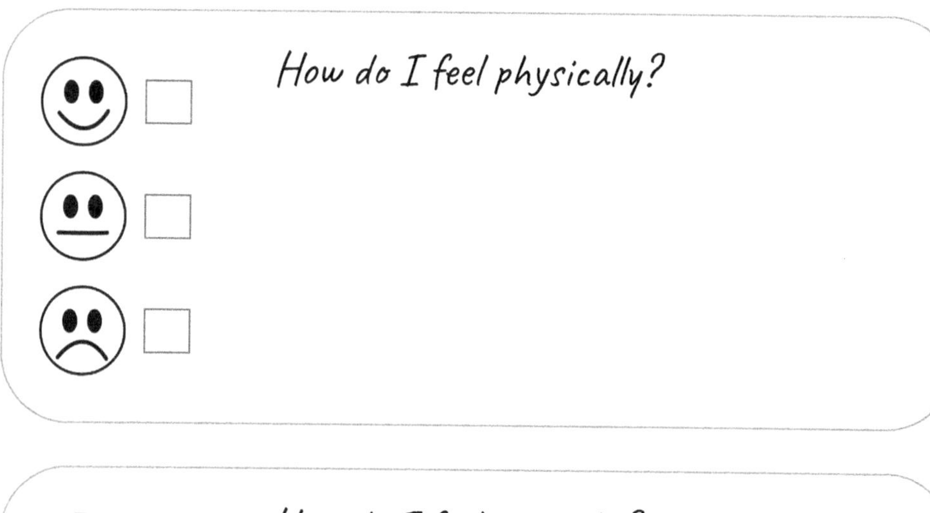

How do I feel physically?

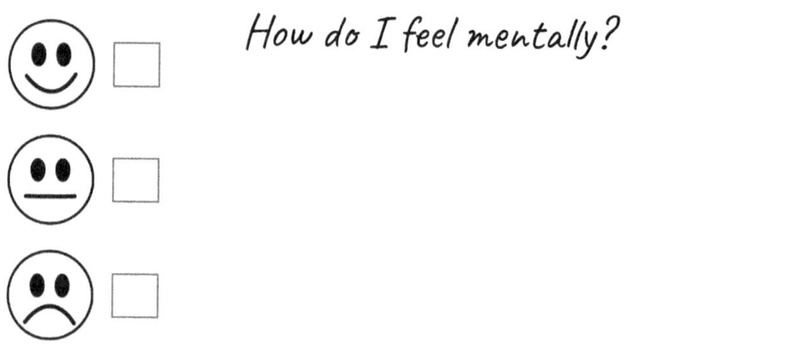

How do I feel mentally?

This week's GOALS

Day 71

Date _______________

breakfast

lunch

snacks

dinner

Workout

cardio ☐ ☐ strength

flexibility ☐ ☐ rest day

zZzz

Day 72

Date _______________

breakfast

lunch

snacks

dinner

Day 73

Date _______________

breakfast

lunch

snacks

dinner

Workout

cardio ☐ ☐ strength

flexibility ☐ ☐ rest day

zZzz

Day 74

Date _______________

breakfast

lunch

snacks

dinner

Workout

cardio ☐   ☐ strength

flexibility ☐   ☐ rest day

zZzz

Day 75

Date _______________

breakfast

lunch

snacks

dinner

Workout

cardio ☐ ☐ strength

flexibility ☐ ☐ rest day

zZzz

Day 76

Date _______________

breakfast

lunch

snacks

dinner

Workout

cardio ☐ ☐ strength

flexibility ☐ ☐ rest day

zZzz

Day 77

Date ___________________

breakfast

lunch

snacks

dinner

Week eleven completed !

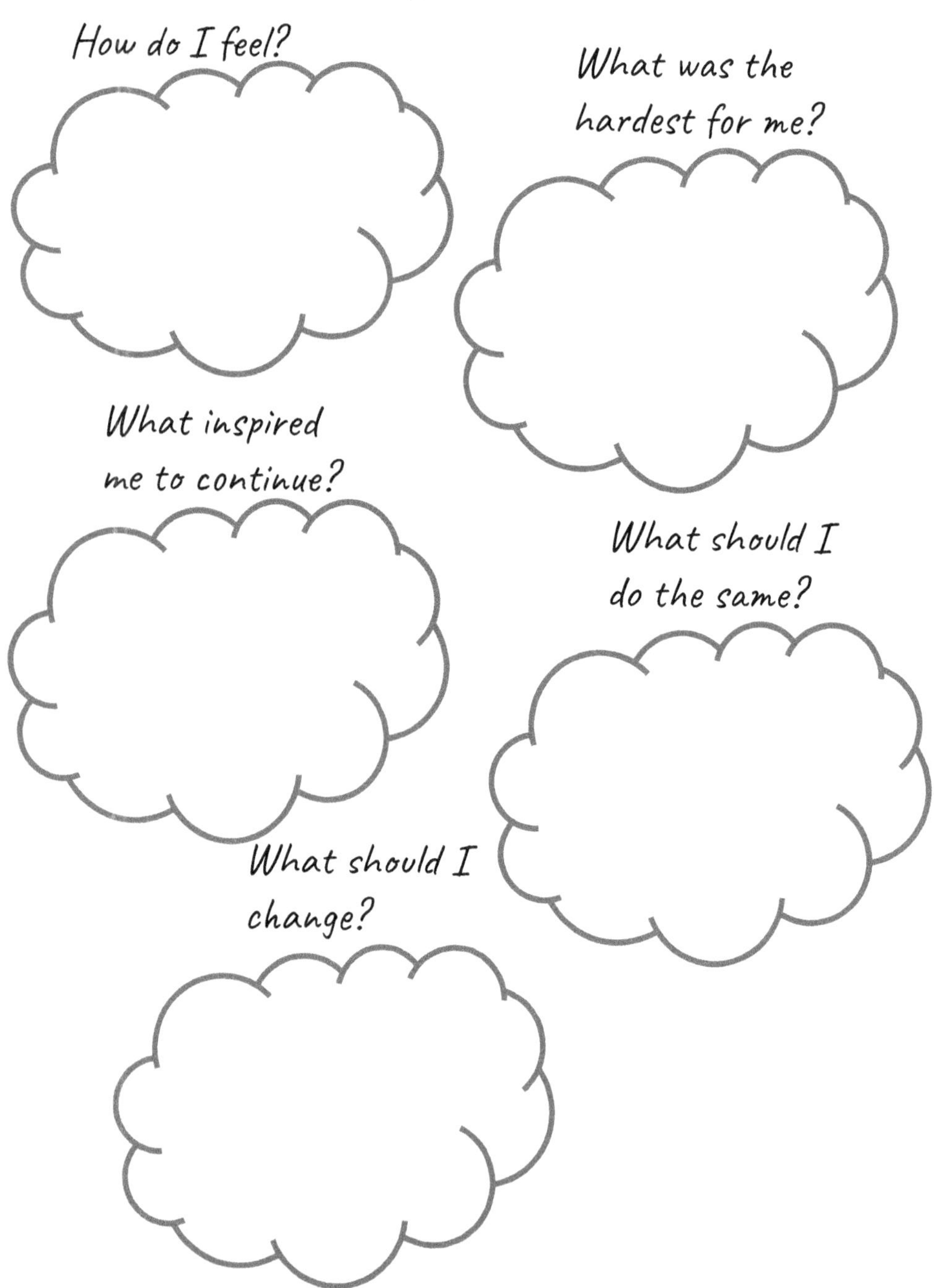

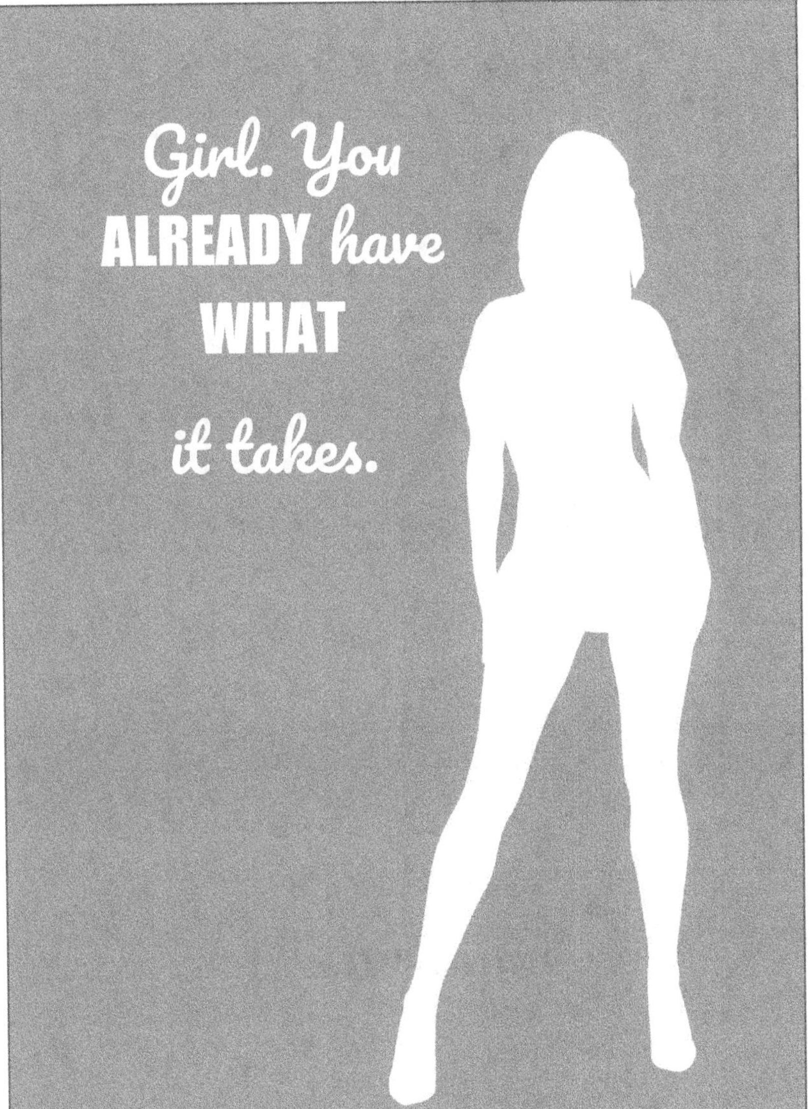

Girl. You ALREADY have WHAT it takes.

Week Twelve

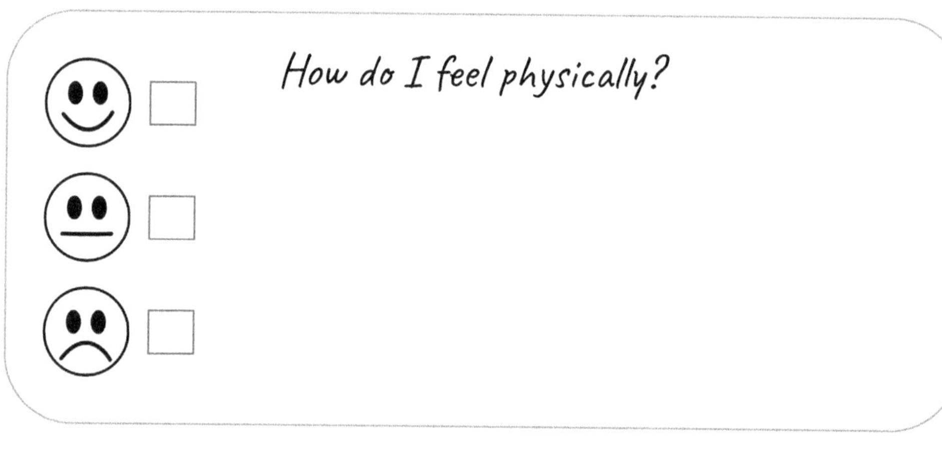

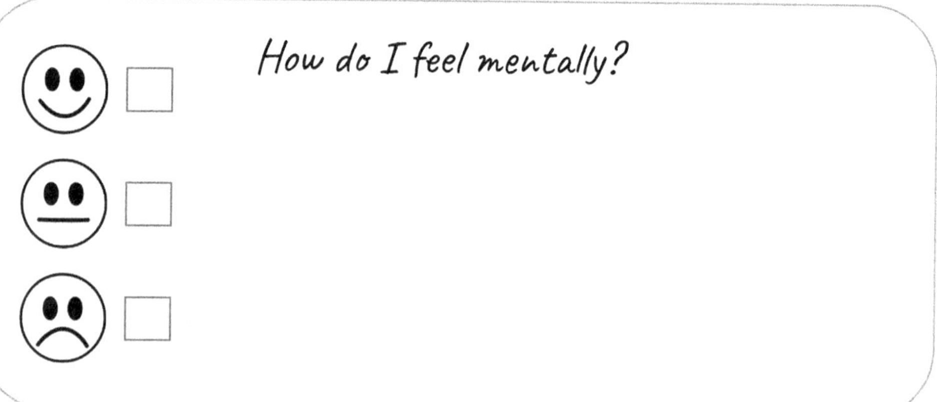

This week's GOALS

Day 78

Date ___________________

breakfast

lunch

snacks

dinner

Day 79

Date ________________

breakfast

lunch

snacks

dinner

Day 80

Date _______________

breakfast

lunch

snacks

dinner

Day 81

Date ___________

breakfast

lunch

snacks

dinner

Day 82

Date ___________________

breakfast

lunch

snacks

dinner

Day 83

Date ___________

breakfast

lunch

snacks

dinner

Day 84

Date _______________

breakfast

lunch

snacks

dinner

Week twelve completed !

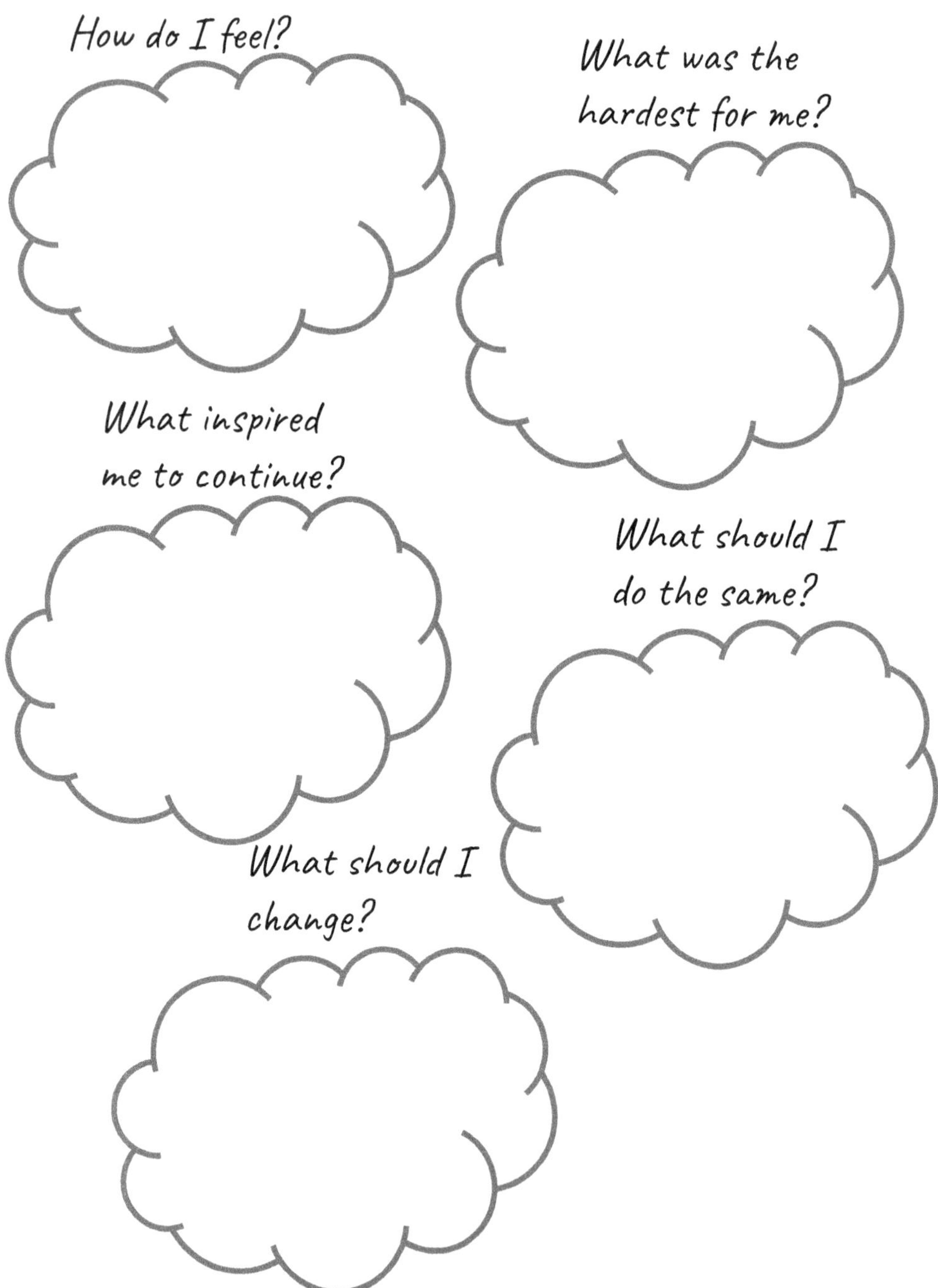

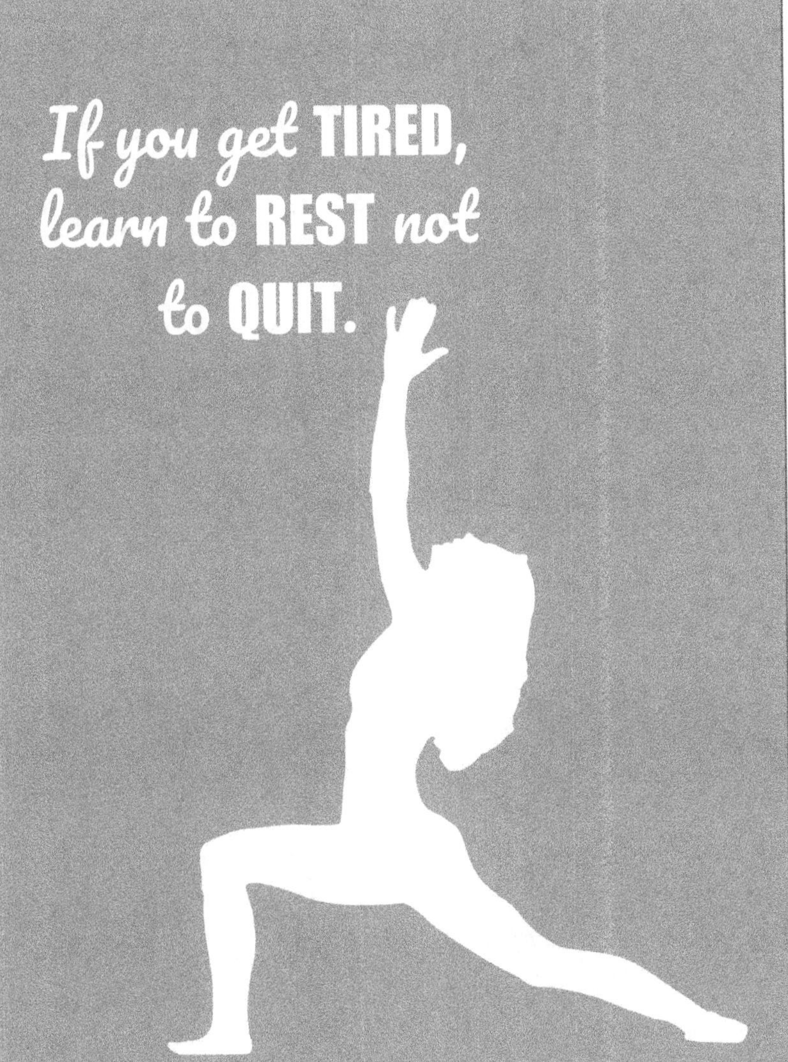
If you get TIRED,
learn to REST not
to QUIT.

Week Thirteen

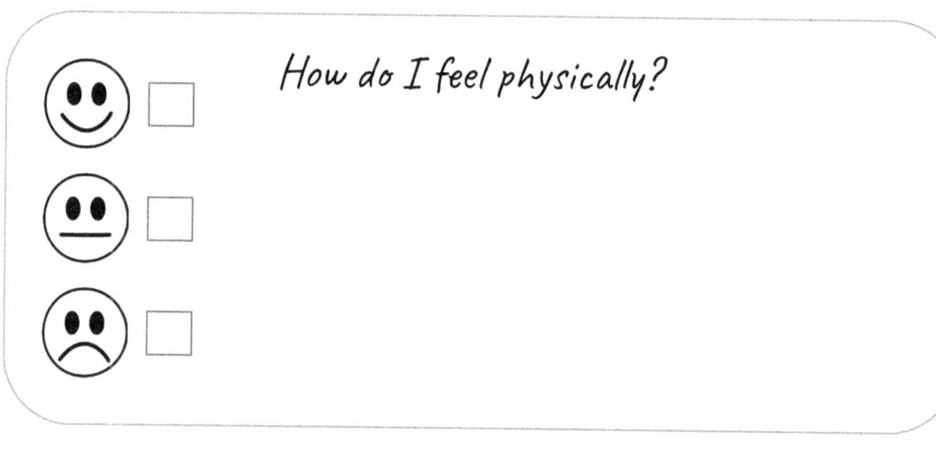

How do I feel physically?

How do I feel mentally?

This week's GOALS

Day 85

Date ______________________

breakfast

lunch

snacks

dinner

Day 86

Date ______________

breakfast

lunch

snacks

dinner

Workout

cardio ☐ ☐ **strength**

flexibility ☐ ☐ **rest day**

zZzz

Day 87

Date ___________________

breakfast

lunch

snacks

dinner

Day 88

Date _______________

breakfast

lunch

snacks

dinner

Day 89

Date ______________________

breakfast

lunch

snacks

dinner

Day 90

Date _______________

breakfast

lunch

snacks

dinner

Workout

cardio ☐ ☐ strength

flexibility ☐ ☐ rest day

zZzz

You did it !!

90 day
challenge

COMPLETED

Take the time to reflect on your experience!

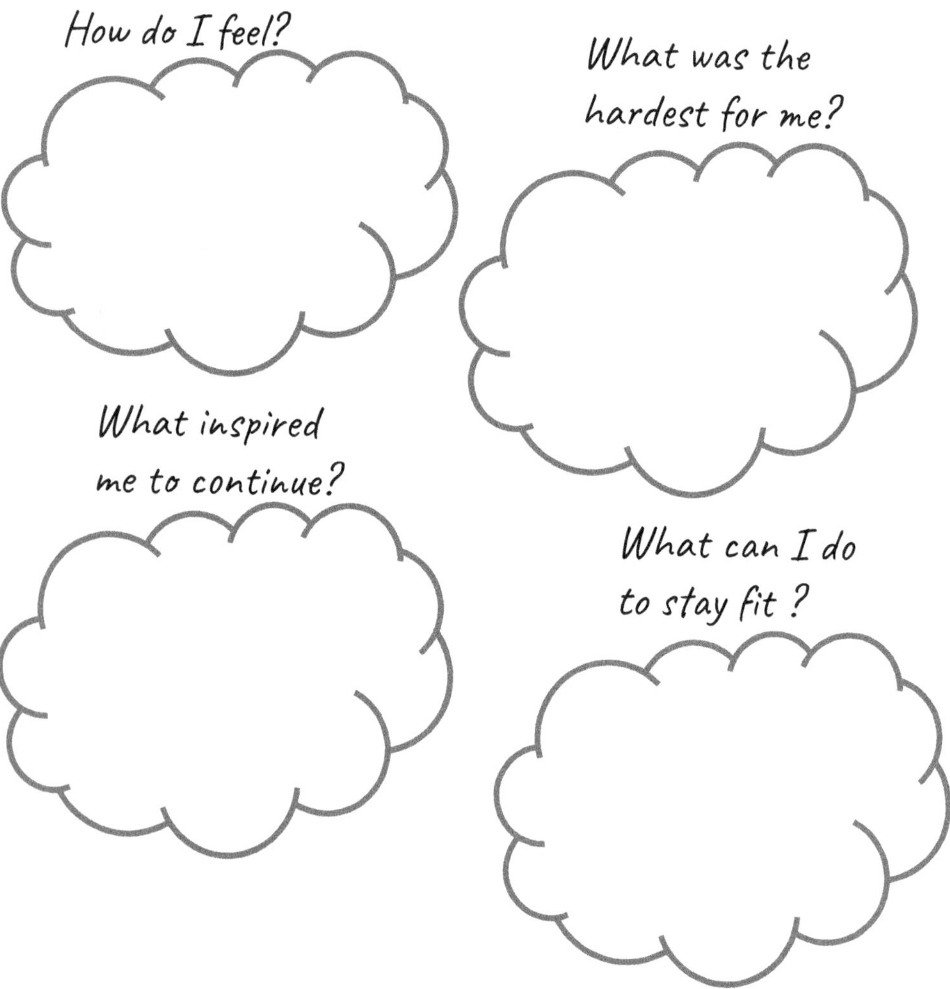

Let's get fit!

Name ______________   Height ______________   Weight ______________

Arm L ______________   R ______________

Chest ______________

Waist ______________

Hips ______________

Thigh L ______________   R ______________

Calf L ______________   R ______________

Finishing stats

finish

Put your new
picture here

Me now! ___________
                date

Remember, it always seems
impossible until it's done.

Stay fit
and get ready
for your next
challenge!